Cancer
&
Me

My Cure My Salvation

Cancer
&
Me

My Cure My Salvation

Patsy McClendon McDonald (Brown)

iUniverse, Inc.

New York   Bloomington

Cancer & Me
My Cure, My Salvation

iUniverse books may be ordered through booksellers or by contacting:

iUniverse
1663 Liberty Drive
Bloomington, IN 47403
www.iuniverse.com
1-800-Authors (1-800-288-4677)

ISBN: 978-1-4401-6171-1 (pbk)
ISBN: 978-1-4401-6172-8 (ebk)

Printed in the United States of America

iUniverse rev. date: 9/14/2009

Book Dedication

I am dedicating this book to my family that means my work family because of all the encouragement that you gave me was really appreciated more than you will never know. To my Church family for all that you have done and are continuing to do. I want you to know that I appreciate you and I am glad to know you'll. I am glad to have you in my life.

To my born to family you have always stuck by me through what never I was going through. I really appreciate your continuing support. There is nothing like a family that sticks by you through all of your problems and all your sickness and pain. A true family knows what to do and say in the time of need. I want to thank all my family for this.

My daughter my only daughter this is especially for you. I love you with all my heart and I want you to know that you are special in my eyes. You have always did you best even when no one else though it was your best. You really have been a hard worker and I want the best for you in life. Remember my daughter do not ever give up on anything that you are trying to achieve always give it your best, do not let no one put you down you are a beautiful person. There is always help around the corner when you need it. It may not be the person that you may want to help you but, mother can not always be there for you. Learn to ask for what you want from people no one knows you are in need if you don't ask my love.

To my oldest son you are so special. You are really a special person you are like a light you brightens up a room when you walk in the room. You have a wonderful family. You did a great job with yourselves and you desire all the credit. I love you dearly.

My youngest son you know you are a special person. You tried to help around the house during my time of need. I didn't even know that you could cook, and I don't think that you knew either until you start cooking me breakfast and sandwiches. Your specialty is breakfast. I love you with all my heart and thank you for all that you do.

To the Love of my life you are a special person, stay the way that you are and let nothing change you. You were always there for me and helped to encourage me to keep going, and I appreciate you for that. YOU have been a live saver for me. You are a very special person to me. You have been there even when no one else was there. You have a great personality and will always be loved by many.

CHAPTER ONE
IS THIS A DREAM?

When I was first diagnose I said to myself this is a dream I am dreaming that I am at the office setting at my desk and the phone rings and it's the doctor and he tells me that my results are positive I have breast cancer. It is all a dream but, do I have to wake up why can't make it all stay in the dream.

I was at my desk. Doing what I've been doing for years, when the phone rings. First, I'm thinking that this is another doctor. But when I answer with my usual "hello", I realize that it's the wrong kind of doctor that I was expecting. Of course, he greets me with the same generosity.

"Hello Patsy," he says his voice stiff. "How are you today?"

Well, I'm not the type of person to complain a lot. If I'm hurting, I try hard not to show it. I put on my happy face and swallow my guilt, "Fine."

"Patsy I have your results from your test," he said, "you have breast cancer.

I will have the clerk to call and set up appointment with you so, that we can take care of this matter right away."

I was devastated, I was scared out of my mind I didn't know what to do, or what to say what was going to happen next.

Why not face this battle, and I knew it would be a hard long battle for me and my love ones. People also don't realize that the people around you are also effective by what ever you are going through, and if it changes your life it is going to make some changes in their life as well.

I know that one day there will be a cure for this disease I hope sooner than later. I never knew that so, many people had cancer until I started taking treatments almost every time I went for treatments the room was full. It was just if though it was some kind of plague that was taking over the earth. How can this be? All these people with cancer some lives with some dies with. That why with this world like it is today you must keep the faith? Because I am telling if you don't have or never had cancer be thankful, and pray that this awful thing never happens to you or anyone that you know. I tell you another thing that I found out is that no matter what no two people is the same I may can bear pain longer and take more pain than anyone, but the next person may be able to do something else better than I can. There are no two people that think and acts just alike, believe me but, of course by now you have probably figure that one out to.

It was faith that kept me when I came out of this dream that I had and when reality hit me I cried and cried because I had heard about cancer know people that had been through the treatments for cancer, and sometimes the results wasn't good. But that is why I am telling you to keep the faith and everything will be alright. Believe me I know it happen to me.

People have reasons for doing the things that they do some out of good faith and some out of jealousy. World is so full of jealous people that it is ashamed one person see someone else doing something and they are so afraid that that person is going to get more than them so they try it. But what people don't know is that what God have for one person he might not have the same thing for the next what my success is might not be your success and what your success is not mines that belongs to you. You can't take someone else blessings.

I tell you people it so, true about what God have for a blessing for one person is not another person blessing you and believe me you can't take another persons blessing. If a person gets some work done and they are charged a price your price for the same thing may be different for what ever the reason. My blessing is not your blessing and your blessing is not my blessing. A good lesson to learn some people wonder how that person how that house for that price when they priced it they probably was told a different price that's is because the Lord had a blessing for that person and it wasn't your blessing your blessing may be something else God may bless you with money instead and that other person will wonder how that he get that money how did he come into that money but I will tell it was a blessing. Always receive all blessing in the name of Jesus and be blessed.

People would get jealous and say how that person got all does cars and that house how did you do and what did he do. The Lord gives blessings as he sees fit. My blessings may be to live a good life even after being diagnosed with cancer and your blessing may be money. Our blessings will not be the same most likely what's for you are for you and what's for me is for me, and I will tell you don't get jealous of anybody be glad that your sister or brother is trying to have something instead of trying to tear that people down.

When I was going to get my radiation treatments every time I laid on the table I would pray to God and say God please heal and touch my body I know that lots of people has been burned from this type treatment but I am asking you to protect and heal my body right now Jesus. I prayed this prayer and I prayed every time I went in there. The first time I went for radiation it was a scary thing those machines was really scary. To watch that beam light beaming down on me I know that light was something that I had never seen. I also knew that it could be dangerous and could be harmful that is why I prayed about it.

Know another thing that I learned while going through this process that if you have a real true friend that friend you will know is really a friend because that person will be with you no matter what. I tell you what I mean by that. A fake friend is only going to be there only while you are able to do the things that they wants to do whether its right or wrong as long as you are able to do for them and what they wants. But, a real friend will be there even when you are down and out and has no way of going and when we are not able to go, a real friend will stick by you and when you are down they will be there to lift you up, they are your true friends and I am here to tell you my dear true friends are very few you can count them on one hand.

So, the best thing to do is to keep Jesus by your side no matter what. Never let him go he will always be there. When you are lying there in pain and there is no one around call on him he will be there for you, and he will never let you down. Remember God is every where even though we can't see him he is there. When you are walking in the spirit you could feel him, you could feel his present there.

I will tell you something else that happened during this time when my hair came out my head was as clean as the back of my hand. When it started to grow back it was like baby hair just like my hair was when I was a young girl. I wonder is it going to stay like this or will it change. That remains to be seen. I am afraid to put chemicals in it, I am afraid that it will come out again. I was wearing wigs but one day I we was leaving for home we, had just stepped out side the building where I work and when we stepped out side the wind was blowing so hard it took my wig, hat and sunglasses right off. My friend that was walking with me went after my wig and hat but, I didn't even bother to put it back on. The day after the wind blew off my wig next day I just said what the heck I will just is wear my bold head. So, after this sometimes I would wear a wig and sometimes I would just go bald and just wear my bald head. There where no reason anymore to be ashamed of my bald head and I am telling you this is something to go through when a women loses her hair, its it frightening most women don't want to be bald especially from an illness. My hair has begin to grow back now, and, I am thankful for that, I will be glad when it grows long right now I have about one inch of hair on my head but I have been wearing my own hair instead of the wigs. But of course this is just a choice that I made you must do what is comfortable for you. If you are uncomfortable with wearing a wig then, just wear what ever hair you have even if you are bald head like I was from the Chemo treatments it doesn't matter just do it don't think about what people is going to stay because people is always going to have something to say, so don't worry just make yourself happy by any means necessary. I mean wearing what's comfortable to you and doing what's best for you, and everything else will fall in place. I you are so, into your boyfriend or girlfriend or just a friend that makes you feel small by making ugly remarks to you by all means you need to get rid of this person.

So, after that sometime I would wear a wig or sometimes I would just go, bald. But, I just wear my hair even though it's not but about one inch long. I enjoy just watching it grow slowing but surely. I know that one day I will awake and it will be full long and pretty I hope. But the thing is that now I am not afraid to be seen in public with my own hair. I am proud of my hair and I am proud of myself for just being me I know that it's really me and who I am. I think that everyone should just try to be their own selves and don't let people influence them to be anything different. That is how a lot of children gets in trouble trying to be like their friends and they don't know like will be better for them if they just be their selves. That is all that God wants for each person to be who he made them to be. You must continue to trust in him in everything that you do.

I have a special friend at work that really believes in me because of her encouraging words it really made taking treatments easier. No matter how we try, we are always going to need each other one way or another. God is everywhere he lives in people. One thing I have always said when God gets ready for you to do something you are going to do it. I think that is when for instance you may go to a car lot to buy a car you know your credit is jacked up but, yet the load goes through.

Do you wonder why that is? When God gets ready for something to happen it happens, he can make them say yes when you know the answer would have normally been no. He has all power in his hands just trust and believes in him and everything will be alright.

Have you never wished for something and the wish came true. Isn't he a wonderful God; he might not come when you want him to be he is always right on time? He will never leave you just hold on and he will bring you through what ever hard time you are having. It is all about trusting in him and believing in him. He will see you through. You can not put your trust in man because they will mess up everything man only thinks of himself and how he is going to make it, don't ever forget about that. No matter how nice a person seem be careful especially when you don't know them because they can take advantage of you for their own befits.

CHAPTER TWO

LET'S BEGIN

My Story
By Patsy McDonald (Brown)

Well, let me tell you how it all begins. I had back surgery last year May 2007 and diagnose with high blood pressure and diabetes three years before that. I thought that all could happen have happen. I also thought that my world as I knew it was about to come to an end.

During the time that I had back surgery this was a bad time I thought but, it turned out that it wasn't as bad as I thought it was. Because the Lord was just getting me ready for another big task, the pain that I suffered at this time was minor compared to the pain that was to come. After my back surgery I was at home for about four months due to the fact that I had to have physical therapy, I wasn't able to drive myself at this time. My youngest son began to learn to drive and he would sometimes take me where I did need to go but, he wasn't able to drive on the interstates so, we could only go local places. But that was just fine, because we still were able to go to church, and to some stores. He didn't have driving license of course he was only twelve at the time. But I thank God for him, and the things he would try to do.

I met the love of my life about four years ago. I did not know at the time that he would one day save my life. One night we where watching T.V. playing like couples do, sitting side by side on the sofa, he gently rubbed my breast.

"Baby, you've got a knot here," he said.

"Oh, stop playing around. I don't have a knot in my breast."

"You do. I'm serious. You need to see about this." He held me tighter.

You talk about being afraid I was because I had people in my family to die from cancer even after treatments. I was so, afraid that this was cancer but, then I said to myself no it can't be, because I didn't feel any pain in my breast for that fact so, maybe its just a knot that will go away.

I have a twelve year old son, I love very much he is the apple of my live how could this happen to me and what do I do. I called my daughter she had a knot in her breast also, she has had knots in her breast before several times and has had to have surgery for them, and was lucky that it wasn't anything as serious as cancer. So, I also had the hope that maybe minds was something like the knots that she gets since after all I was her mother maybe she got this terrible thing from me. We both made appointments with Mississippi Breast Center, LLC Breast Surgical Oncology Clinic in February 12, 2008 which was a day before my birthday. So, when that date came I met my daughter at the clinic. She had been there before so, after we signed the book in just a few minutes they called her name and she went back, I was still filling out paper work because it was my first time visiting the clinic. After I finished my paper work I carried to the front desk walking slowing in fear. Almost like if I knew what but, still hoping and praying that this would be good news not bad.

In a few minutes they called my name, as I was entering into the hall way I bumped into my daughter.

"I am okay," she said, sighing with relief. "The doctor said he'll see me in August."

So, now it was my turn, "Mama, do you want me to go with you?" Her worry caused frown lines to appear between her eyes.

When I went to the back the doctor felt the knot in my breast and he said I need to do a biopsy on it. So, he did, and he looked at it on a machine like a sonogram. He said this don't look good I am sending you to the Women's hospital for more tests right now. So, I got dress and took the slip of paper that the clerk handed to me, and my daughter and I went to the Hospital which was next door. They did some tests and I went back to the doctor's office and he told me that as soon as he got the results we would let me know.

I was scheduled for a breast mammogram on February 18, 2008 and for an MRI, CT, and Bone Scan on February 27, 2008. I'm here to tell you this was also something that was scary to me because I never had a CT and Bone Scan before. The receptionist was very nice and so, were the nurses so that went pretty smooth. I tell you the Lord is always working over time. In everything he does he is always right on time he knows what he wants to happen and when he wants it to happen. The Lord puts people in certain places for reasons and sometime it is just to help another person or to just enlighten someone's day. But for what ever the reason only he knows, but one thing is for sure I know that he knows best.

Some days after that I was at work and my phone rang it was the doctor he told me that the tests where positive I had breast cancer. I cried so, loud that one of the ladies that work with me came and carried me to the bath room, and I was there for a while crying out loud, I couldn't help it. This was the worst thing that could never had happen to me I thought. I had heard about chemo and radiation and how bad it was and what it could do to a person and how it effects the body Oh Lord why me I said Oh my God why is this happening to me. When I made it back to my desk I called some family members to let them know what the news was that I had just received. I am here to tell you just was the worst thing that could happen to me I thought. But I met a lot of good people, my doctors where the greatest. I had good nurses and all the staff was good to me, like I was telling you earlier God put people in certain places for reasons and only he knows why or what he intend for that person to do.

CHAPTER THREE

TALKING ABOUT BACK PROBLEMS

I had told you earlier in this book that I also had back problems. Well I was in a car accident sometimes in August, August the 29, 2008 to be exact, with the problems I already this started my back and it started back acting up worst than it was, so I went backs to the doctor that treats my back. My appointment to see this doctor was on the same day that I had my MRI of course they set it up for. January 09, 2009 I went to get an MRI, the lady at the front desk she was very nice and everything, she say go and fill papers out and sign where you see the x mark, and so I did and I went to the window and she said your insurance is still with the state, I answer yes. She made a couple phone calls and told me that my deducible was five hundred and my co pay was two something she said that leaves you a balance of seven hundred and something dollars. I looked at her and I laugh and stop playing with me lady. We both laughed because she knew what that meant I do not have any money.

She was going nice but, I will pay it but, it will have to be on payment terms. Everything is so, high. When I was younger and I use to hear people say that they had insurance I thought that the insurance will pay for everything in full, because you are making monthly notes to have insurance so why can't they pay for the full visit. Hey something is wrong with that picture. What do you think is wrong with that picture? Hey I tell you making monthly notes you should pay even if you job pays fort your insurance still somebody is making the notes on it. Somebody need to re look at that situation. Then you have the car insurance the same thing if you have an accident they go to talking about a deductible I really don't think that this is right you are paying them every month to have this insurance making monthly payments that should be deductible enough not like you are going to have an accident every day.

I went and sat down, and then in a few minutes they called me to the back. The young lady that did my MRI she was so nice. What did I tell you earlier I been blessed like that to have some that really care on my Health take care team. This is a blessing because some of these people don't care if you are comfortable on the table or not they are just trying to do their part so that they could go home for the day or just so they can finish what ever it is that they need to finish. That's why I can tell you that it matters I have had MRI and was uncomfortable they say you'll be ok it will only take a minute but, just young lady said lets get comfortable, is this comfortable to you, and I really appreciated that more than anything, especially when you are already hurting and don't feel good you really need to be comfortable. So, she gets an A+ in my book.

After I finished she was walking me back to the front and she said this is your cd with pictures of your back on it, it is your to keep but, if you have to pick up another we can make another but, it will cost you something. After I left there I had an appointment with my doctor for my back, when I made it I signed in, the people that works there is really nice to, but remember I told you that I was blessed like that to have all nice people that cares about their job. My thing is how you call your self in a profession working with people and you don't to work with people and you are not a people person if that be the case that would be the wrong job for that person. I will tell you there are lots of them out there. Believe it or not and you can tell who they are just as soon as you make it through the doors to be treatment that attitude lets you know very quickly believe me. Well when they called me to the back I talk with the Nurse first, and then a few minutes after the doctor came in. We looked pictures of my back and he explained to me what the problem was. He decided that since there is nothing in the lower part to separate the disk that I would need an injection this injection would have to be preformed by another doctor so, we will have to set up an appointment for this so, now I am waiting for this doctor's office to call me with the appointment. He also said that if that don't work we can fix it by doing surgery and insert a screw in my back which will be an adjustable screw. But we will try the injection first and if that don't work we know what we need to do next. Well if its not one thing its another that what most people would say or they would call it bad luck but, you have to realize things just happen and it not bad luck or anything like that. Things wear out just like clothes wears out but, you can always fix it. The only time you can't fix that is death. But as long as you lave breath in your body any that arrives or any thing you can fix it believe me. If you boy friend or girl friend leaves you can fix that and have self convenience in yourself and everything will work out. Don't forget what I told you about people that low rate you, baby you don't need that, and if you are that in love with person and they are low rating check this out what do you think that means, I will tell you they are trying to bring you down so, that you can be more dependent on they and they also think that you won't leave them because this is the way they are controlling you be stronger than that if they love you it wouldn't be any name callings. You can talk to a person without calling them out of their even if you is angry with a person or your mate; there is no need for disrespect.

Your back plays an important part with your body. You can not walk, or run without your back so, you what to do what you can to keep it in good shape. So please do what you doctor tell you and keep in mind what he tells you so, later you will remember, because when you are feeling better you may forget and try to lift something that you shouldn't

Young ladies and means that why when my next book come out you must read I will tell you more about relationships and to control it better. Knowing the key is the answer it is always a way to handle a situation believe me. But, remember you don't have to be disrespected no one should disrespect the other.

The funny thing is if you find someone else that person that was doing this entire name calling him or she would suddenly change but, like I say that will be a different book that was just seek per view. I will love to be on a talk show, I believe that it is hard to do. Maybe because they are so busy because it is so much going on in the world to cover. I told you something good can come from something bad but, I tell you something else I will still be around until they find a cure for cancer because brothers and sisters I will not ever give up not ever and my advice to you is to do the same no matter what the situation is.

Once you have a problem with you back and you get operated on it is a life time thing and you will never be the same, don't lift this don't pick up that, if you know what I mean. You can't lift thing pick up things like you did before if you do you will mess up believe me because I still would try to pick up my little grant nephew I love him so much but, now I know I can't do that, that is a no, no once you have back surgery some people don't realize that, but it is up to you to take care of yourself because remember some of them is not going to care as long as what they need is being met so, listen to what I am telling you. It is all about taking care of yourself believe me if you do that everything else will fall in place because how could you help someone else if you don't first help yourself. No one is going to care for you like you so, if you know you have had back surgery you already know that the doctor has already explained to you about lifting, so don't do it. You can help someone in another way, other than to hurt yourself. You remember you will be the one going back under the knife they may set and wait for you to return after surgery but, you along will feel the pain so treat yourself right and do the right thing.

Now your life will be changed for ever and ever, all the things that you used to do as far as lifting is over, the heavy containers that you unused to could pick up and throw over your shoulders, is over. Picking up the heavy wood for a fire is over, unless you want to go back and have another surgery, because that what will happen if you mess things up by lifting what you shouldn't.

CHAPTER FOUR
TALK ABOUT CHEMO

On March 05, 2008 I was scheduled to see the Oncologist so that I could start Chemo therapy. I saw my Oncologist on March 05,2008 my family was with me my oldest sister, my daughter, my nephew, my son, and my baby sister, thank God. Well we talked with the doctor for a minute then she said I need to take a look will everyone leave out, and they did. She said I can shrink this tumor, then she called everyone back in the room and we set up the first day of my Chemo treatment which started a new chapter in my life. We decided to start on March 15, 2008 which was on a Thursday I choose this date because the doctor had explained to me that with my chemo I would need a shot the day after to kind of help put some things back that chemo will take away. So, on Fridays I would have to come back and get a shot. I also knew that I would need for someone to take me for these treatments, the love of my life jut happens to be off on Thursdays and Fridays so, this would work just fine great so this was the plan.

The doctor also told me that I would be doing 8 weeks of chemo therapy, then I would have surgery, then it will be followed by eight more weeks of chemo therapy and after I finish with that I will be doing 32 treatments of radiation.

I had surgery on March 06, to have a port inserted in order for them to administer the chemo through so, that we wouldn't have to use my veins. This was very helpful in the long run.

Well when March 13, 2008 came around it was time for me to go and get that first treatment of chemo; I bet you I dragged around that house as long as I could try no to go. But as time pass by I know I had to go and do what I needed to do. I love my son and I knew I wanted to be around for him. My love told me he said baby you know you got to go, so please don't be trying to talk your way out of going. Come on he said its time to go you're are going to have us late. So I got my purse and headed for he door late of course I was scared half out of my mind I didn't know what except really, I hadn't never did this before. I asked God for the strength to carry this through.

So, it took us about an hour to make there, to the place. When we arrived my oldest sister, my daughter, my youngest sister, and my nephew was there. We was late so, everyone was looking at my love because they thought he was the cause but I later told them the truth it was me, I was scare I was dragging around. I didn't know what to do I took my time taking my bath; I walked as slow as I could. I found other things to do; I even decided the dishes need washing, and the house needs cleaning. I'm sorry, So, I signed in at the desk, and in just a few minutes they called me to the back my love went with me to the back and wow I was really about to go out of mind by this time. The young nurse got to insert the butterfly into my port and I screamed it was still tender from surgery but, it was ok I just afraid of needles. So I asked them to ask the doctor to give me something for the next time so, I wouldn't feel it. So, after they inserted the needed we went back up to the front, and the next time they called my name I it was to start injecting the chemo, and now here comes they called me and we went to the back and they had me to sit in this reclining chair all nice and comfortable then they inserted his bag of chemo, by sticking the needle into the butterfly needle that they had left inserted in my port in my chest. Almost immediately after just a few minutes my stomach started to hurt I told the nurse she said you shouldn't be hurting I told her but I am please give me something and she did. I felt to sleep. In a few hours I was finished. When I went to desk I asked for my dates to changed I wanted to get the Chemo on Fridays and the shot on Saturdays. So that is what they gave me. That Friday My love carried me for my shot I will tell you that shot sting like a bee and the chemo made every bone in my body hurt I had never felt so much pain in my life.

There was times when I felt like if I went to sleep I wouldn't wake up to see the next day and I would think about my son my baby boy, and I knew I had to get the strength from somewhere. My son was so, great he would fix my breakfast in the mornings before I go to work, and I don't even know how he knew to do this or that this needed to be, but that little fellow never ceased to amaze me. I thank the Lord for him he is great. I studies his books he is an honor roll student he always try's to keep that every since he started school he has been a honor roll student, he attends Morton Middle School but, of course they have great teachers and this is also a blessing they cares about their students and they want their students to grow in faith and in the world he loves his school and his teachers and this makes a big difference when a child attend school and the teachers as well as the principal cares about the students and cares about what happen to them, that is so good because you know that you don't have to worry all day long about your children because you know the school officials' cares and they will do what ever necessary to keep the children safe.

I decided to continue to work during this process so I took the papers that my job human resources had gave to my doctors to fill out and I carried them to my job. My work family was very good to me they let me work around the treatments. They were so wonderful. My church family called me to check on me. All of this is what helps a person to keep going it is so wonderful to have a good born to family, work family and church family I am so blessed thanks to the Lord. I am so blessed.

So, the next time I went for my Chemo my love carried my on Friday s and my oldest brother carried me for my shots on Saturday. People don't realize what they have until it's gone and it's too late. Always tell the person that you love that you love them everyday don't wait until something happen and then tell them you tell them everyday so, that they would know because you don't know if you are coming back the next day or the same day and you don't know what is going to happen to that person that day or the next day. So, this is a habit that I do, I tell my love ones that I love them that way if something do happen you have stated how you feel about that person or persons.

So the time came for the second round of Chemo. My love carried me for my Chemo and I was so, glad to see my oldest sister, my nephew he is so special to me, my daughter who is always there even when I didn't want her to be. This was great I had the best support group. After getting my chemo which always takes a little while we headed back home. Saturday morning my oldest brother came right on time I knew to be ready because he don't play around if he say 7:00am that exactly what he means. We made to the building, as soon as I signed it in just a few minutes they called my name. I went to the back but since it was just a shot it didn't take long just a few minutes and I was headed back to the front. My brother looked at me and he said "did you get the shot"? I said yes I got the shot. He said are you sure you got the shot that sure was quick I say yes I got the shot he looked at me again you got the shot. I had to take him back to the back and find that nurse that had gave me the shot so that she could tell him yes she got the shot. That was the funniest thing to me. He said well you came out so fast I just wanted to be sure this is nothing to be playing around with.

This is my oldest brother he would do anything in the world for me, he wanted to make sure that everything was o.k.

When we were small we were close and we are still close now. He always wants to take care of me the best that he could. So, I expected questions from him, and believe me he wanted them answered.

I remembered the doctor telling me that my hair was going to fall out in about two weeks of taking the chemo, but I decided that I was going to be smart. I just won't comb my hair I will just pull it back into a pony tail maybe that is why the other people hair came out they combed it. So, this work for a few weeks, then one day I was sitting in the bed watching television and I rub my hands over my head and all my hair peeled back like an orange. I couldn't believe this, it look like a wig when you hold it up in the air. It took it and put it in a zip lock bag. I'm going to keep this for souvenir; I had never seen anything like this all of this was new to me. I continued to work while I taken my treatments with the ok from my job and doctor. I was so, blessed, I was a great deal of pain all the time, I would wait until after I get to work to take my medicine and this still didn't stop the pain and when I look back on it I don't know how in the world did I do this. I know it was all the Lord no other way.

One day I was at work and I was hurting so, bad, I couldn't do nothing but put my head down and couldn't help but, to cry and I felt hands in my back it was my co workers rubbing my back, their support really helped me and kept me going at work and help to give me the strength to continue. I know that I had bills to pay and a son at home there was no way that I needed to be off work I didn't have disability insurance. It was my own fault every time the insurance people came by year after year my friend girl would tell me Patsy you really need to take that insurance you never know what may happen, I didn't listen to her. I didn't take that insurance because I believed I was healthy, that I didn't need it. But I know now that disability insurance is vital for everyone. While I may never again have a need for it, I would have had it to help out during this time.

Well now I was at the point that I didn't have no hair on my head and every time I looked in the mirror I felt worse I was bald headed. But one thing that I had did when I first found I had breast cancer I went that day and bought me a wig I knew it would be hard for me knowing and seeing myself without hair on my head. So, I started to wear my wig this was a beautiful long blonde wig. But it was a little too long, so when I got to work I asked one of the young ladies that work with me to cut it some and she did it was so pretty I was blessed there too, the young lady carries a lot of great talents. She did a wonderful job on it.

CHAPTER FIVE
COMFORT FROM OTHERS

It was another young lady that worked with me that was also diagnosed with breast cancer a few months before I was and she had been through some of the things that I was going through I had several talks with her she was a great encouragement to me during this time and still is. This was another blessing. She told me lots of things that I didn't know and I would like to thank her for it. She is a very wise person and I thank the Lord for her.

My director she is a very understanding person no one could have a better person for a supervisor than she. She is a very special person. She's understanding in all that she could be. By the way I told you that I was blessed.

I would never forget the day I came into the office and I spoke with her and her director about my illness, and her director say we will work with your schedule and they both worked with my schedule for my treatments, I thought the world was coming to an end but, help was just around the corner. This meant more to me than they never will know.

During the time of treatment my Oncologist gave me several prescriptions among them was a numbing cream this helped a lot with the injections. I just put in on at least one hour before treatments and put a large band aid over it this numbed the area before hand and made the injections so much easier. This really helped me alone with my chemo treatments. I never lost my appetite I took vitamins everyday. This helped my body to stay strong. I ate plenty of fruits and vegetables. I drunk lots of juices this also helped my body to stay strong and wealthy. I tried to do everything right such as eating and drinking. I drank plenty of water. Drinking lots of water help to keep fluids in my body and helped to keep my body flushed.

The chemo treatments made my body weak, and I was in lots of pain. I did a lot of praying and remember I had my work family, my born to family and my church family how could anything go wrong. As time pass by my first set of chemo treatments was finally over.

I saw my oncologists at least every two weeks she would check me and talk to me and see how I was feeling, and also I would tell her if I needed anything. I met my reconstruction doctor May 14, 2008 it was time to set my appointment for my surgery. So he and my cancer doctor would set his appointment. So my surgery was set for May 20, 2008 I made it to the hospital that morning our pastor, my baby sister, my daughter, my nephew, my love and in law was there. I had a lot of support. I went into surgery to get the remainder of the cancer tumor removed, and reconstruction work done. In a few hours I was out. My friend from work came by to see me I was glad to see her she is a special friend. Also my friend that has been a friend for years came by to see me it was such a up lift to see my family and friends and to know that they where thinking about me on this day. My people from my job called to check on me. This was very encouraging to me. All of this was great for me. All of the great words of encouragement and the visits was great for me and helped to help keep me going on.

After I had surgery it was eight weeks before I went back to work I was cut from breast to the other. During surgery the doctor found out that I also had cancer in the lymphoid as well. But, he said that he got it all I was grateful for that. I had the best doctors and the best team for this, I believe in my heart. Thanks to God for all he has done for me and my family. My neighbors sent money, food and would help with anything that was asked another blessing from the lord I had good neighbors too. I was so blessed and still is blessed the Lord has been good to me and my family. After surgery I had to drain bags hanging on each side it had to be empty and measured every day my love did that too. I also had home health coming to check on me too. Home health came until the drains were taken out. One of the drains stayed in for two weeks and the other one had to stay week longer because it wasn't ready to come out. The right side the side that the cancer was in took a little bit longer. After I saw my cancer doctor and reconstruction doctor in June I was to start Chemo treatments again. My Oncologist told me that this set of chemo was a little different it will not make me weak but, will give my body lots of pain, and she was right. Every bone in my body was hurting, for days and days I was in pain. I made sure I took my medication and tried to eat like I should. All of this was very important in the healing process. I started chemo treatments again on June 20, 2008; I had to go through eight more weeks of pain that will never end, to me. This will take lots of prayer and lots believing which I have always believe in God, and I knew that he would protect and keep me, this I knew my pastor of our church kept in touch and always say call me when ever you need me. Just the words of encouragement was good all the people at church my church family was very helpful. It is so, good to have a good church family remember a family that prays together stays together. My oldest sister and my nephew were there for all of my treatments they where so great. My oldest brother took me on Saturday s for my shots and when he couldn't make or had to work my cousin would take me for my shot on those days. He was a blessing also. Yes him, he is a man and I am blessed to have him as a cousin. He doesn't know up to this day how grateful and thankful am about that because he didn't have to do it. He took the time out of his day to carry me for treatment. You know when a person do something for you be thankful because no matter what or how small it seems to you, it is something big because it takes time out of a day for person to take you some place or do something for you they could be doing something else but, instead they those to do something to help you, and you also know that in Gods eyes this is a blessing to you, and this person will also be blessed, and we always give thanks, for that.

This was the worst thing that I thought that could never have happen to me. But I know that the Lord those everything for reasons, he has his own reasons maybe it was so that the story could be told in a different way so it could be understood about the strength that we can endure and the trust that we must have in the Lord in order to make things work like it should in our lives.

There was times that I was afraid to go to sleep because the pain was so intense that I felt that if I went to sleep that I would wake up to see the next day. Everyday when a woke up I was so happy to see this new day. I was glad to be living. Even though to look at my face you wouldn't know that pain that was in, and how I was suffering. Each day was a challenge for me just to get up and tries to get to work or anywhere was a task. Because of the fact was everything I did I did it while in pain. I can't speak for others and how it was for them but, I can only tell you what happen to me. Even today my legs and arms still pain and hurt, and I really don't understand why. But the main important thing is that I still live.

I had some wonderful neighbors during this time some cook, some gave money, and some took me places when I needed to go. Lots of time there were things that needed to be done and I tell you I was more than happy to get the help. I can understand now how to live with pain it is all about knowing Christ and living in the Lord. There will never be a perfect person because the perfect one is all gone but we all can be the best that we can be in Christ.

It was the funniest thing I looked the perfect picture of health. You couldn't just look at me and tell that anything was wrong. I had the will power and still have the will power and it will never leave me. This is my blessing, and my strength it all comes from the Lord. This was a blessing that he bestowed upon me, for myself to have and to keep. You know the Lord bless each of us as he sees and only he know why what happens and what ever happens. It is he that gives me the strength to keep going. I blessed me with this talent to know how and what to do to keep on going no matter what comes and this is what you have to do for yourself and never mind what anyone thinks because it is all about you and you keeping the faith in yourself and in the Lord and he will carry you through I know just ask me.

Finally my eight weeks was over it seem like it was forever and forever thank you Lord I just want to thank you Lord. My son sometimes would cook for me. Sometimes he could fix me breakfast, or lunch my baby son he is really neat. I really appreciate everything that he done for me. He was great. My love my would call me and ask me do you want me to bring something so, between everyone I was fine. All of this was a blessing and I appreciate everything that everyone did for me.

CHAPTER SIX
RADIATION BEGIN

I met my radiation doctor on July 30, 2008; the whole crew was so nice they are really the best. He met me my oldest sister and my nephew met me there. The doctor explained to me everything that he was going to do, and he also told me what to expect. He was really great; the whole team I am telling you was wonderful. They worked with me in everyway.

This doctor was great and the team I had with this radiation is great.

I had to do thirty two treatments of radiation. Everyday after I left from treatment I would mark and R in red on my calendar this would let me know that I had completed treatment for that day and I looked forward to the next day because everyday that pass was one over and complete and behind me. During this time my cousins with Chicago came to visit me at different times but they came I really enjoyed them both. I was so excited to see them. We really had fun this help me to forget about the things that was going on. I continued work all while I was taking my treatments my job was so wonderful. Believe me when I say my job was wonderful I mean it; I couldn't have done it without them. This is my work family, there are different kinds of families, work family, born to family and church family it takes them all to make one life whole and I am telling you when all of your family is wonderful and works hard to make things right you could not ask for anything more than that.

Everyday when I make it to the building for my treatments I come through walking as fast as I could because I know I was just making right on time and sometimes late. So, I came down the hall, sometimes I hear them say there she comes. I would run right into the dressing room change as fast as I could and I heard one them say she is just like wonder woman.

Every week once a week I would see my radiation doctor he would check me to make sure I was getting any burns or peeling skin. It was so funny when he first my telling me about some of the side affects he told me that I might get burn or skin may peel. I looked at him and said none of that is going to happen to me. No matter how often he tell me that I would tell him none of that is going to happen to me.

The thing about is that I really believe that I had faith in him and in the Lord, and I knew that the Lord wasn't going to let this happen to me. My faith was just that strong and guesses what none of that happen to me. Everything turned out just fine.

The Lord was always is always with me and others. Holding on to that belief was what got me and keeping the faith once I have it. The Lord will never say no, you could always call on him he might not come when want him to but, he is always on time.

Life is just like magic it could be here today and gone tomorrow I have seen lots of people come and go this last year, and I wonder what is this world coming to when I look at television and there you see mother killing her own child. People shooting each other and I say to myself why what in the world could they be thinking about. Life is precious and you only get one chance at life but must live it to the fullest but always in Christ. See the world, even it that mean from a book or from television as long as you see it for what it is, and always remember it don't take but one time to do sometime but, once its done you can not take it back you can ask forgiveness for your wrong doing but you can never take back anything that you have done. If you ask God to forgive you for doing something, you should try not to make the same mistakes over and over again. I think that what's wrong with us today we will ask forgiveness and go back and do the same thing over and over again.

I worked during my process and treatments I was determined that I was not going to let this get me down, by no means, and I didn't. This the way I would like to see any one that is going through this does, keep strong no matter what and no one said it was going to be easy and it's not. I will not tell you that it is easy because its not. My love for my children was one of the biggest things to help to keep me going. I love them all. I also have grand children, that I wanted to keep seeing, and also would like to watch him grow up and I knew that if I let go and just let myself leave this earth I wouldn't see them in this world again.

I would wonder on the nights that I couldn't sleep I would lie there and wonder if I don't wake up what would happen to my children they needs me, especially my youngest. I don't want anything to happen to him. He's a great person with good potentials. Cancer is like a snake it eases upon you and before you know it, it got you. I am going to continue to fight this battle and I will not give up. If it never happens to you remember do not give up and continue to fight. As long as you are fighting to live because that is what it is like fighting each day to live to see the next day and taking each day one day at a time. This is all you can do and when you have done this you are fighting your battles never let anyone talk negative to you that will be the devil trying to make you let go so that he can take over and if you let that happen then he has won. So always continue to fight for your life because this is what it's all about.

Patsy McClendon McDonald (Brown)

Everyday I told myself yes I can, yes I can I can do this no matter how bad the pain is I know I can do it. I was so glad when Christmas came, and really didn't think that I was going to make it to see Christmas 2008. But, the will power to live that burns inside of me say yes you will be here.

CHAPTER SEVEN
DEALING WITH THE SITUATION

You know I would like to reach out at many people as I could in order to help someone even if I could just help one person I have did a lot. Understanding pain is a hard thing do, but, learning to live with pain is also a hard thing to do. Just remember that your doctors are your health line, keep them in formed with everything that is going on with you, and that way they can make the best decisions for you and your body, before you take any type of medicine or go to a dentist always consult with your doctors. Because during the time of treatments there may be some medicines that you may not be able to take only your doctors will know this so, make sure you inform them of what's going on with you and believe me they will know what you need rather than you just taking anything over the counter without being sure.

It is very important to let your doctor know before taking any thing some medicines don't do well when taken with others. I know you are thinking it's just an aspirin or it is just Tylenol always ask your doctor to make sure it is safe you don't need a reaction from medicine because you have been through and going through enough.

Another thing I did when they call to the back to draw the blood they always draw blood each time you go because they run all types of test to make sure everything is ok. When they call you back the second time it is to start the procedure of injecting the Chemo into you. I had a port in my chest for this so, they insert something like a butterfly needle into my check, and they have a nice big reclining chair for you to lie back in. Immediately after my chemo starts I would send my friend to get me something to eat, this was the funny thing because no matter how bad the taste was I never stopped eating even if it tasks like rubber I still wanted to eat I guess I would call that being greedy, but I knew that I needed to eat no matter how it taste or what it looks like as long as it was healthy. During this time I ate a lots of fruits, vegetables and drank plenty of water, one of the key factors is to eat but, also drink plenty of water during all of your treatments this is very important. Remember they will give you materials to read about your conditions, and they do have helpful things, in them.

But if you are hurting anywhere or any place during your treatment let your doctors know sometimes there are things such as pain pills they can give you to help with this pain, but I don't know why the pain pills didn't do much for me, but every body is different, and it doesn't hurt to try.

Don't forget when you are taking Chemo treatments, or getting any type of treatments that involve getting a injection also ask your doctor for some type of numbing cream because this will help you as far as getting the injection you follow the instructions but, the type that I had I put it on, I mean put it on thick in the area that you know that they will be using and put a large band aide on it that holds it and make it adsorb in your skin better. I put it on one hour before I leave for the doctors office for my injections, I 'm telling you do all and any thing that will help to make it better for you. You are the one feeling the pain and not on one else knows the pain that you are going through. Support groups are good if that's what you want you can do the support groups but I didn't because I didn't want to hear anything negative, all positive because I was going through enough already, I didn't need anything negative in my life, you always want to think positive and be positive if anyone come to you talking anything negative you really don't need to be talking to them.

I had a lot to happen to me in such a short time but, that is ok things happen and we learn to live and deal with help from the Lord and he puts people in our lives in order to help us with the things that we go through. I really believe that even when I was trick out of the money for the room it was for a purpose, this person was probably going around doing this to people and on one ever turned them in at least by this it will put a stop to his tricks on people.

Somebody has gotten to be the one to turn this person in so that he won't go around tricking other people out of their money especially the older people that would be probably like me, didn't know, but now learning don't trust anyone to get into your wallet like that. One thing that they do is keep on for money until it's all gone then you doesn't see them any more. Why is people like what do they accomplish can't be much because soon everyone knows about them, and know not to use them then their business gets smaller because they don't have customers and they wonder why, well it's the way you conducted your business that's why, and people talks and the word get out do not hire this person because he's bad and his work is terrible. It is good to put things in writing but, if you put it in writing someone is going to read it and it will help someone out there, there is someone out there that need theses words believe me it was a time when I needed words of encouragement but there was no one to give it to me, that's why I'm writing this book as a word of encouragement for anyone out there that needs it. It's all in the book that's what I always say.

The reason why I wanted to write about this was to give encouragement to someone else that may be in need of encouragement during what ever hard time a person may be going through. If I can give some encouragement this is what I want to do. I know that there are people out there that need this encouragement. There are so, many people out there that are going through the fight for some illness and need a word of encouragement. I am happy to be able to write this book that I may help that someone.

Always stay lifted up no matter how bad the pain is, this was my way of keeping a life because you, know when you in a lot of pain and the pain continue constantly sometimes this will make you want to give up and let go, and leave this earth. This pain is worst that having a nail driven through your foot or should I say stepping on a nail. It is worst than having a baby. There is nothing that can describe it because I have tried to put it in a prospective or know what is was like to be in this pain, but even I wasn't able to label it, because it was the worst pain that I had ever been in because it was a continuously pain that didn't stop until weeks after all the treatment was over so, therefore you had months and months of continually being in pain, and even today my legs, arms and back hurts so, bad that sometimes it is hard for me to walk on my legs. But I will never give up and I am intending to be one of the ones that are here when they finally find a cure, I am telling you; you can do it, if I can do it anyone can.

I wanted people to know that you can get over anything if you put in the effort to do and the time. Even though you may be in pain you can work through Chemo treatment and radiation, but it will take a lot of effort, because this is a painful process even though the doctors don't even realize how painful this is for a person. We are grateful to them for the knowledge and know how that the Lord has provided them with, but I am telling knowing how to deal with pain is another story, it takes a lot of praying and commitment to what is going on with you, and then you make the decision that nothing is going to stop you from doing the things that you need to do in your life this is the decision that I made and I am proud of this.

What do you think about a book with such few chapters well let me tell it don't take one hundred chapter to tell what I need to tell you but, it may take another book believe me it is more blessing to give than to receive and I want to give you all the information that you need to make it in this life I will share with you all my experiences but, like I say it will be in the next book. This is a book about encouragement and to give you encouragement. Always believe in yourself other people will always try to put you down and most of the time when a person is trying to put down on another person that person what to be just like the one that he's putting down. So watch for that. Sometimes people will pretend to be your friend but, all the time they are trying to set you up for the big fall. You must be very careful it you all the sudden start to do good and people start to gather around you try to remember was this person there before you was doing good was this person my friend before he or she needed something or did they just look and though you where doing good and decided I need to be friends with her or him.

Most of the time you can count your friends on one hand, the real friends is the ones that I'm talking about not the fake ones that just appeared into your life when they though you was doing well. Your real friends has been there all the time. Your fake friends only appear when they think that you are doing good or maybe you can help them. I'm here to tell you about the real friends are there all the time even when things are going they are still right there by your side.

I also want to tell you if you have a lover, boyfriend, live in friend or what ever you want to call them, if they low rates you all the time calling you out of your name such as fatty, ugly or anything like that baby you don't need them you can do bad by yourself you do not need help to do bad believe me you are a beautiful person, and that person knows it, but to keep you a stein low he or she calls you names and this will keep you also under their power because you would think oh don't no body want me because I am ugly and fat. But baby this is not a true statement you are beautiful and there is a woman or man that's is looking for you to be there mate and they will treat you like a king or queen believe you don't have to take that coming from anyone find you a place to go get a apartment if you don't have a job get you a job. I am telling you things are better than they look or seem, I have been through this is and I know my someone used to let me know all the time that I was old but tell you one thing I wasn't old anymore then all of the things where different, so pay them no attention when they say things like that but, also remember you don't have to take. I know that you want the person that you love to just love you back and be that person and lover that you want him or her to be but, remember it don't always work like that and most likely if he or she is calling you names it is time to let it go. When this starts to call you names, most likely he or she is seeing someone else or doing something that they shouldn't be doing one or the two, but remember you can do bad all by yourself you don't need no help in that department.

Most men's will try to have control over your mind just so, they can take advantage of you and some women let the young men talk them into having a babies but I am here to tell you he is not going to treat you any different just because you are having his baby, now he knows that you will be in his life for ever and a day because you have connection his childe now look what you did. Now you got a child to take care of and plus your self and he has went on by his business and met someone else to get pregnant but, that ok you still can fix that, you can still get a job and take care of your baby put your little friend on child support do other wises he will soon forget that he has that baby over there and stop giving you anything to help with that child. But like I say that another story girls just to let you know what ever the problem may be it can be fixed one baby two babies, three babies or four babies what ever the number is we can fix that we can get a job and put these men's on child support and help our selves there is nothing to big or small for the Lord he will give you strength to do this.

One thing I hate to see is an unsure man that try's to bring some young lady down just because he's down instead of fixing his problems and bring his self back up. You must keep uplifted in Christ and keep uplifted spiritually with your body, soul, and mind and there is nothing that can take this away from you not nothing.

CHAPTER EIGHT
LET'S GET COMFORTABLE

During this time I also that would be a good time to make myself comfortable so, I decided that since I didn't have a bath room in my bedroom it would be a great thing this would make things more easier for me. So I decided to get a load to do an addition to my home, this will be a bedroom with bath and of course a closet. I put in for the load when I first got out of the hospital from having surgery, but didn't get it until sometime in August. I got the loan and I didn't really know who I was going to get to build that room. So, I asked around and this particular person recommended this person that I had got which didn't do a third of the work but before I knew it I had completely paid plus over paid one thousand over the cost that we had contracted it for. The contractor just kept coming back saying he needed more material money. So one day I told him there is not more money this was in October. I tell you he didn't come back to do any thing else he just dragged around every time I would ask him when are you going to finish the room he would come and do a little something, never completing then one day I realized I had been tricked he wasn't going to complete he had just trick me out of my money. He would always say I am waiting on the plumbing but I am here to tell you even if he was waiting on the plumber it was plenty he could have been doing because none of the outside was complete this man had only completed about one third of the this work. Then one day I called I asked him when are you coming to complete this room he said I am waiting on the plumber so, I called his plumber and his wife answered the phone, and I asked her is your husband going to complete the plumbing work at my house she said yes he said that was will complete but he still sick I told her he been sick for three weeks. I got to thinking after I put the phone down and I called the plumber back and his wife answered the phone again I told her to tell him that he didn't have to come I would get someone to finish and have a blessed day. I tried to call the contractor back but, he didn't answer his phone so, I text message him to let him know his services was no longer needed due to the poor quality of work. Because by this time I had really look at this work that he was doing the walls was uneven floor, uneven the little panel that he did put up had to be taken back down because the walls was so, uneven. How could anyone do anyone like this? But I guess it was easy I wasn't going to be able to really go out there and check everyone so he took advantage of that, I am telling you this to let you know don't trust no body not even your friends when it come to money people will look out for their selves and forget about you. You must only trust yourselves when it comes to money. Because I will still have to pay for this loan plus pay someone to redo what he did and plus compete this job.

It is something how people takes advantage of people for their own needs. The old contractor that I had hired was that type of person but, I didn't know it. The person that gave me his name probably knew it or probably didn't I really don't know. You know something people tries to help people the best that they know how but sometimes your best isn't good enough with some people because they will not appreciate it.

I end up getting the same people that put my heating and cooling unit in to take the job of completing this room for me which we are still in process of getting complete due to it being in such bad shape from the first contractor. He really messed up that little that he had done. But, this goes without saying don't trust people even some people that are supposed to be your friends because people most of the time looks out for their own interest then yours interest last. Because I am telling you this man work was so, terrible it's reason way that he had many jobs that part was a joke I bet he didn't hardly have any jobs and was glad to find another person to trick, I sure that everyone knew about him except me. You know look like to me instead of going around tricking people he would learn to really do the jobs he would come out a whole lot better. After this big mess he made at my house then people began to tell me about him, and of course after I got trick out of my money but, I hope that you know what to do in that case, you take that person to court because this is fraud, you turn them in to the BBB and to the licensure broad because you don't want them to continue to do people like this, because nine out of ten it will be either the elderly or someone that's ill that's not able to go and actual check this person out. So let me tell you I am doing just the things that I just mentioned to you I am going to try to make sure that this doesn't happen to anyone else by this person. I don't see how a person could do something like this and live with themselves but, I am learning some people do things like this for a living, and sometimes people like this probably been going around for years doing this same thing just but no one probably turns them in so, they continues to do it. But, not me if a person does something that wrong like this they must be turned in so, that this person can't do another person and just continue on with the same trick.

I later found out that even the second person that I had hire wasn't any better in some ways than the first. He wasn't picking up all the materials that he had claimed to be either, even though I was paying for it all and still have my receipts. I even found out that the Air Unit that he had placed in my home in which I had paid him for and have receipts wasn't hooked up correctly and he had left a lot of things unfinished, but, had received the money for it.

It is so, much that I wanted to tell you about it will probably take another book. I will have another book coming. It is so, much about living that people needs to know and something's are just for knowledge. You know a lot of things I didn't learn until this year, but I thank the Lord for letting me deal with everything in the way that he did. When someone tricks you out of your money, and especially when you taken a load out for that money you must remain a Christian and just let the laws and rules of the law handle it.

Not only that I learned that my walls was uneven, concert floor uneven the ceilings was also uneven this first person that I had hired to do the addition on to my house didn't care and didn't know how to do anything he was just all a fake, and everyone needs to know about him so, that they would know when they see him not to get him to do any thing because he don't know how to do anything correct he could do it, but it wont be correct, you would end up getting someone else to finish and do corrections. I found out also that the roof was leaking and that something else to have a leaking roof on top of everything else. But, the people that are working on it now will also have to repair that. This room is costing me more that I anticipated for it to be what started out to be a small project became a large project, due to the mess that was made by the first person that I hired to do the job, so, let me tell you always check out a person and check out their work don't be in a hurry, because you also need to ask around to see what type of work this person do, and not how is his or his business personality but also how is the company and this person work.

I also wanted to tell you about my younger brother he is a preacher, he can really tell a good message and I love to hear him because he really explains what he is saying so that even the elderly and younger people could understand. I visited his church today it was all good. Before he got his church I had already joined the church that I am attending. But I still make a point of visit his church because I want him to know that I love him and I want him to continue in the right path as he is doing. He has a great family and I am glad for him. My older brother also has a great family they are in church and that's a good thing. I am proud of my brothers and their families. My sisters are great they have their families and they are also in the church we all attend different churches. We all are trying to stay in the Lord. A family that pray together stays together always remembers that for your household. But you know we have always tried to do the old ways. One thing I could tell you about the elderly they are very knowledgeable and could tell you a thing or two, if you just listen. My grandmother used to tell me about the old days and I would listen to her every word because I knew that there was no better way than to her it from someone that had really been there. The elderly they are so, knowledgeable in this world really the words of wisdom comes from our elderly.

My baby sister keeps my mom, in other words my mom lives with my baby sister. She has so much to do I wouldn't dare ask her to do anything else when I was ill because she had enough to do already, and know one knows that when you have a person living with you that you have to take care of like that it changes your whole life. You can not go where you want to go, and you can do what you want to do, it changes everything about your life, even though some people looks at it like its nothing but, let me tell you it is a big difference in you are keeping someone for life than when you are just picking them up for the weekend or for a couple weeks. Because when they are living with you, you have put up with attitudes and believe the elderly can have some attitudes because they know they can't do the things in live like they used to and this is a upsetting thing to them, so sometimes they takes it out on some one else and that's usually is the person that is keeping them and that is a bad thing because this sometimes makes a person think well, is this all in vine no it isn't in vine because you are helping a person that would have been in the nursing home if it wasn't from you, and I tell you something that you may not believe but, some people actually does better in the nursing home than they do at their relatives home. There really are some good places out there but, they all could be good if we would keep check on our elderly like we should but, you know that you can't always be there and that's understandable, just be there when you can as often as you can. Believe me your parents understand more than you know.

CHAPTER NINE
THE LAST RADITATION TREATMENT

I had my last treatment of radiation on September 18, 2008. I was so, happy and the team that was giving me my treatments was happy to we was so happy and they was so happy for me we all was hugging each other my oldest sister, and my nephew was there that day also. They had a gong button they said do you want to hit the gong I said yes it was just like on that T.V. show that used to come and it sound loud like it too it was fun. See there are lots are great things that came out of this I met lot of good people and they met me. It taught me to be strong in everything you do, see from the being of my treatments to the end I had to fight for my life from that day on. It was a battle to get up and do anything I had to put forth more afford because I was in pain, and I will tell you to get up and go to work that wasn't easy. But it knows that the Lord let it happen for a reason maybe I can help to encourage someone else by telling my story. I tell you something else too it helps when you are being treated by people that cares about people, I was so lucky I had the greatest team of doctors, and the greatest staff of people giving me my treatments I was so blessed. I thank God everyday for what he has done for me and I will never get through thanking him for what he has done and for the distance that he has carried me.

Having a great team like this was wonderful I know that this was also God's work he put together a great team for me one thing he knew I was already afraid, so again he stepped in and did the job, and I thank him for that. I have always believed in God and this is a great encourager for everyone, because he will always be present even when our friends are gone.

I can say this over and over again I had a good work and doctor team, with during this treatment. All my doctors where so, good, they took the time out with me and my situation and made it all work, I am so thankful to them for everything that they have done for me through the Lord Jesus Christ that gave them the power and the knowledge and the know how to put it all together and know actually what they need to do, and how much to give me and when.

Everything that we go through in live is a challenge for us, and it teaches us about our strength that we have within our selves, body, sprit, soul and mind. This is a enter Sprit with God that will give the extra strength that we need when our body and soul is in trouble, that means such as illness, or spiritual sometimes we just need a spiritual blessing, and this comes from the Lord.

During this time I met the owners of an air heating and cooling company that installed my air and cooling unit at a reasonable price. They were very good and they stand by their work. You can't find people in this world that you could trust like that to let in your home and they do a job and not try to get over on you. These people are the greatest at what they do and they care about people and they don't try to take advantage of people like some people do.

They came in and installed my heating and cooling system at a reasonable price, and the price they gave me was the price that they installed for. You know some people will try to beat you out of your money especially if they see that you are vulnerable, what I mean by this is that you don't know the prices of things or ill and can't really check behind them to see what they are doing, so they quote you a price for one thing but, install another because you don't know the difference. You really have to watch people because the must of them really don't care they just be trying to stay a flow themselves so, if they over charge you are install something that cheaper than what you paid for it doesn't matter to them. But, these people are on the up and up, they are great and I highly recommend them to anybody that needs any type of work done. They not only do heating and cooling I can do about anything that you need.

I pray everyday and I thank the Lord that I am still here, and everyday is a beautiful day to me. If anybody asks me how I am doing I am doing fine and it's a beautiful day that is what I would say because it is a beautiful day to me. I know could not have been here, but he spared my life and I believe in my heart that he did this for a reason. I believe that he wants me to tell about so, that it may help someone else in some way form or fashion. This January we start two thousand and nine. This is a new year and we must try to do better this year than we did last year, and I am not say try to make a New years revaluation I just say try to do better every year than you did the last year no matter what it is, and it could be something small that you want to accomplish it so, let do it.

Even thought I am finished with chemo by injections and radiation. I will still have to take a chemo pill for five years. This is also something that is different for me. This pill makes my bones hurt. Sometimes my legs hurts so, bad that I can hardly walk on them at this time I pray harder in order to keep going. If you haven't been through anything like this it is hard to explain and its hard to understand only those that has truly been through this type of pain knows exactly what it is about, we all can imagine. I know some people that just given up instead of fighting, at this time you must fight

I have fought and will continue to fight the battle of cancer if I can win this battle so, can you be strong and always keep Jesus in your life, he can fight and win any battle for you, just call on him, and he is always there. He was there for me.

www.ingramcontent.com/pod-product-compliance
Lightning Source LLC
Chambersburg PA
CBHW061218280526
45784CB00006B/2543